Love Your Yoni

A Comprehensive Guide to Caring for Your Yoini

By Dr. Ava Eagle Brown

CEO of His & Her's Haven-

'Taking Care of You' in Santa Cruz- St. Elizabeth

Disclaimer:

The information presented is the author's opinion and does not constitute any health or medical advice.

The content of this book is for informational purposes only and is not intended to diagnose, treat, cure, or prevent any condition or disease.

INTRODUCTION

For the purpose of this book I will refer to the yoni as Yoni as my favourite word for the V spot.

The yoni is a crucial and complex organ that plays multiple essential roles in a woman's life. It is not only a key component of the reproductive system but also contributes to overall health and well-being. Here are some reasons why the yoni is an important organ for a woman:

Reproduction: The yoni serves as the birth canal, allowing for the passage of the baby during childbirth. It is a vital part of the reproductive process, facilitating fertilization and supporting a growing fetus during pregnancy.

Sexual Pleasure: The yoni contains a rich network of nerve endings, making it a highly sensitive and pleasurable area. It plays a significant role in sexual arousal and pleasure during intimacy.

Yoni Lubrication: The yoni naturally produces lubrication during sexual arousal, which helps reduce friction and discomfort during sexual activity.

Yoni Microbiome: The yoni has a unique ecosystem known as the yoni microbiome. This collection of microorganisms helps maintain a healthy acidic environment, preventing the overgrowth of harmful bacteria and infections.

Menstruation: The yoni is the exit point for menstrual blood during a woman's monthly menstrual cycle.

Self-Cleansing: The yoni has a self-cleansing mechanism, where it produces natural discharge that helps flush out bacteria and dead cells, maintaining a healthy balance.

Indicator of Health: The appearance, smell, and feel of the yoni can often be an indicator of overall health. Any changes or abnormalities in the yoni area may signal potential health issues that need attention.

Given the yoni's critical roles, it is essential for women to prioritize its health through proper hygiene, regular gynecological check-ups, safe sexual practices, and attentive self-care. Empowering women with knowledge about their bodies and yoni health allows them to make informed decisions and maintain their overall well-being throughout different stages of life.

So the question many maybe asking why write a book on yoni care.

Writing a book on yoni care serves as a valuable resource to educate, empower, and support women in taking charge of their yoni health. It contributes to breaking down taboos, reducing stigma, and promoting a proactive and holistic approach to women's well-being.

Writing a book on yoni care serves several important purposes:

Education and Awareness: Many women may lack comprehensive knowledge about yoni health and care. A book on yoni care can educate and raise awareness about the importance of maintaining a healthy yoni environment, normalizing discussions about this vital aspect of women's health.

Empowerment: By providing information, practical tips, and self-care strategies, the book empowers women to take charge of their yoni health journey. Empowered with knowledge, women can make informed decisions and seek appropriate care when needed.

Addressing Taboos: Yoni health has often been shrouded in taboos and cultural sensitivities. A book on yoni care can help break down these barriers, encouraging open and honest conversations about women's health.

Supporting Transitions: Women go through various life stages that can affect yoni health, such as puberty, pregnancy, menopause, and aging. A comprehensive book can address the specific needs and concerns of women during these transitions.

Reducing Stigma: Some yoni issues, such as infections or discomfort, can be stigmatized or misunderstood. By providing accurate information, the book can reduce the stigma associated with certain conditions and promote a compassionate approach to women's health.

Holistic Approach: A book on yoni care can emphasize the importance of adopting a holistic approach to women's well-being, taking into account physical, emotional, and mental aspects of health.

Encouraging Proactive Healthcare: Regular gynecological check-ups and self-examinations are crucial for early detection and prevention of potential issues. The book can encourage women to prioritize their health and seek timely medical attention.

Providing Practical Guidance: The book can offer practical advice on choosing suitable products, practicing safe sex, managing menstrual care, and nurturing yoni health during various life stages.

 vi

Table of Contents

Note: This comprehensive guide is intended to provide general information and guidance on yoni care. For personalized advice and medical concerns, it is essential to consult a qualified healthcare professional.

Chapter 1

Understanding Yoni Health

The yoni is an essential part of the female reproductive system and plays a crucial role in sexual health and overall well-being. Understanding yoni health is fundamental for every woman to maintain a balanced and thriving intimate area. In this chapter, we will delve into the anatomy of the yoni, the yoni microbiome, and common yoni issues and their causes.

1.1 The Anatomy of the Yoni

The yoni is a muscular, tube-like structure that connects the external genitalia (vulvto the cervix of the uterus. It serves multiple functions, including facilitating sexual intercourse, allowing menstrual blood to flow out, and acting as a passage for childbirth.

Key structures of the yoni include:

The yoni canal: This is the inner part of the yoni that stretches and contracts to accommodate various activities like sexual intercourse and childbirth.

The yoni opening: This is the external opening of the yoni, located between the labia minora.

The cervix: The lower part of the uterus that protrudes into the upper end of the yoni canal.

1.2 The Yoni Microbiome

The yoni microbiome refers to the community of microorganisms that reside in the yoni. These microorganisms, including bacteria, yeast, and other microbes, play a crucial role in maintaining yoni health. The balance of these microorganisms is essential for preventing infections and maintaining the yoni's natural pH level.

Lactobacilli are dominant bacteria in a healthy yoni microbiome. They produce lactic acid, creating an acidic environment that helps protect against harmful pathogens. Hormonal changes, sexual activity, menstrual cycles, and the use of certain products can influence the yoni microbiome.

1.3 Common Yoni Issues and Their Causes

Several factors can impact yoni health, leading to various issues. Some common yoni problems and their causes include:

Yoni Infections:

Bacterial vaginosis (BV): An overgrowth of harmful bacteria that disrupts the natural balance of the yoni microbiome.

Yeast infections (yoni candidiasis): Caused by an overgrowth of the fungus Candida albicans.

Trichomoniasis: A sexually transmitted infection caused by the parasite Trichomonas yoniis.

Yoni Discharge:

Normal yoni discharge: A healthy yoni produces a clear or white discharge that varies throughout the menstrual cycle.

Abnormal discharge: Changes in color, consistency, and odor may indicate infections or other underlying issues.

Yoni Dryness:

Often linked to hormonal changes, such as menopause, that lead to reduced lubrication.

Certain medications, stress, and immune system disorders can also contribute to dryness.

Yoni Itching and Irritation:

Allergic reactions to certain products (e.g., soaps, detergents, feminine hygiene products).

Infections or skin conditions like eczema and psoriasis can cause irritation.

Understanding the anatomy and microbiome of the yoni, as well as common issues and their causes, provides a solid foundation for maintaining optimal yoni health. In the following chapters, we will explore effective strategies for yoni care, hygiene, and ways to address specific concerns to ensure a happy and healthy intimate area.

Chapter 2

Maintaining Good Hygiene

Maintaining good yoni hygiene is essential for promoting overall yoni health and preventing infections. Proper hygiene practices help to keep the yoni area clean, balanced, and free from harmful bacteria and irritants. In this chapter, we will explore the best practices for daily cleaning, choosing the right cleansing products, and tips for bathing and showering to ensure optimal yoni hygiene.

2.1 Proper Daily Cleaning

Regular and gentle cleaning of the yoni area is crucial for removing sweat, bacteria, and other debris that may accumulate throughout the day. Here are some tips for proper daily cleaning:

a. Wash with Warm Water: Use warm water to cleanse the external genitalia (vulvand the surrounding area. Avoid using hot water, as it can strip the skin of its natural oils and cause dryness.

b. Use Mild, Unscented Soaps: If you prefer to use soap, choose a mild, fragrance-free, and pH-balanced cleanser specifically designed for intimate use. Avoid harsh soaps or body washes that contain perfumes or dyes, as they may cause irritation.

c. Front to Back Wiping: When wiping after using the toilet, always wipe from front to back to prevent the transfer of bacteria from the anal area to the yoni, which can lead to infections.

d. Pat Dry: After cleansing, gently pat the yoni area dry with a clean, soft towel. Avoid rubbing, as it may cause irritation.

2.2 Choosing the Right Cleansing Products

Selecting the appropriate cleansing products for your yoni care is essential. Here are some considerations when choosing the right products:

a. pH-Balanced Cleansers: Opt for products that are pH-balanced to maintain the natural acidic environment of the yoni, which helps protect against infections.

b. Avoid Douching: Douching disrupts the natural balance of the yoni microbiome and can lead to various yoni issues. It is best to avoid douching altogether.

c. Natural Alternatives: Some individuals may prefer using natural alternatives for yoni cleansing, such as plain yogurt or apple cider vinegar diluted with water. However, it is essential to consult with a healthcare professional before using any home remedies.

2.3 Bathing and Showering Tips

In addition to daily cleaning, proper bathing and showering practices are crucial for overall yoni health. Consider the following tips:

a. Shower Daily: Taking a shower at least once a day helps to keep the entire body, including the yoni area, clean and fresh.

a. Avoid Prolonged Hot Baths: While a warm bath can be

relaxing, avoid prolonged exposure to hot water, as it may lead to dryness and irritation of the yoni area.

a. Choose Breathable Underwear: Wear cotton or other breathable fabric underwear to allow air circulation, which helps prevent moisture buildup and reduces the risk of infections.

a. Change Wet Clothes Promptly: After swimming or exercising, change out of wet clothes quickly to prevent moisture retention, which can create an environment conducive to bacterial growth.

By following these proper hygiene practices, you can maintain a healthy and balanced yoni environment, reducing the risk of infections and promoting overall comfort and well-being. In the next chapter, we will discuss menstrual care and the best practices for handling your period to keep your yoni clean and comfortable during menstruation.

Chapter 3

Menstrual Care

Menstruation is a natural and essential part of a woman's reproductive cycle. Proper menstrual care is crucial for maintaining good yoni hygiene, comfort, and overall well-being during this monthly process. In this chapter, we will explore the best practices for choosing the right menstrual products, menstrual hygiene practices, and addressing menstrual discomfort.

3.1 Choosing the Right Menstrual Products

There are several menstrual products available, and choosing the one that suits your needs and preferences is essential. Here are some common menstrual products and their characteristics:

a. Menstrual Pads: Disposable or reusable, menstrual pads are worn externally and absorb menstrual blood. They are available in different sizes and absorbencies to accommodate various flow levels.

a. Tampons: Tampons are inserted into the yoni canal to absorb menstrual blood internally. They come in various sizes and absorbencies and are an excellent option for active individuals.

a. Menstrual Cups: Reusable and eco-friendly, menstrual

cups are inserted into the yoni to collect menstrual blood. They offer a longer wear time and can be a cost-effective option in the long run.

a. Period Panties: These specially designed underwear have built-in absorbent layers to manage menstrual flow without the need for additional products.

When choosing a menstrual product, consider factors such as your flow intensity, lifestyle, environmental impact, and personal comfort.

3.2 Menstrual Hygiene Practices

Maintaining good menstrual hygiene is essential for preventing infections and maintaining yoni health during your period. Here are some menstrual hygiene practices to follow:

a. Change Products Regularly: Regardless of the menstrual product you use, it's crucial to change it regularly to prevent bacterial overgrowth and odor. Follow the manufacturer's guidelines for usage and change frequency.

b. Wash Hands: Always wash your hands with soap and water before and after handling menstrual products to minimize the risk of introducing harmful bacteria.

c. Personalize Your Routine: Adapt your menstrual care routine to your individual needs and preferences. For example, if using a menstrual cup, you may need to empty and clean it more frequently during heavy flow days.

d. Disposal: Properly dispose of used menstrual products according to local waste disposal guidelines. For reusable products, clean and store them appropriately between uses.

3.3 Addressing Menstrual Discomfort

Menstrual discomfort is common and can range from mild to severe. Here are some strategies to address menstrual discomfort:

a. Pain Relief: Over-the-counter pain relievers like ibuprofen or acetaminophen can help alleviate menstrual cramps. Always follow the recommended dosage.

b. Heat Therapy: Applying a heating pad or taking a warm bath can provide relief from abdominal cramps.

c. Stay Hydrated: Drinking plenty of water can help reduce bloating and discomfort during menstruation.

d. Practice Self-Care: Engaging in gentle exercises like yoga or meditation can help manage stress and promote overall well-being during your period.

By following these menstrual care practices, you can ensure a comfortable and hygienic period experience while maintaining optimal yoni health. In the next chapter, we will explore sexual health and safety, providing valuable information on safe sex practices, contraception, and ways to enhance sexual pleasure while prioritizing yoni health.

Chapter 4

Sexual Health and Safety

Sexual health and safety are crucial aspects of maintaining a healthy and fulfilling intimate life. Understanding safe sex practices, choosing the right contraception, and prioritizing yoni health during sexual activities are essential for overall well-being. In this chapter, we will explore the importance of sexual health, recognizing and preventing sexually transmitted infections (STIs), and ways to enhance sexual pleasure while ensuring yoni health.

4.1 Safe Sex Practices and Contraception

Practicing safe sex is vital for preventing unintended pregnancies and reducing the risk of sexually transmitted infections. Here are some safe sex practices and contraception options to consider:

a. Condom Use: Condoms, whether male or female condoms, are highly effective in preventing both pregnancy and the transmission of many STIs.

b. Long-Acting Reversible Contraceptives (LARCs): LARCs, such as intrauterine devices (IUDs) and contraceptive implants, offer long-term contraceptive protection without the need for daily maintenance.

c. Birth Control Pills: Oral contraceptives can be an effective option for preventing pregnancy when taken consistently and as prescribed.

d. Dual Protection: Combining condoms with another form of contraception, such as birth control pills or IUDs, provides dual protection against both pregnancy and STIs.

e. Regular Testing: If sexually active, regular testing for STIs is essential, especially if you have multiple sexual partners or engage in unprotected sex.

4.2 Recognizing and Preventing Sexually Transmitted Infections

Sexually transmitted infections (STIs) are infections spread through sexual contact. Early detection and prevention are essential to protect your sexual health. Here are some key points to consider:

a. Regular Testing: Regular STI testing, especially if you have new or multiple sexual partners, can help identify infections early and prevent their spread.

b. Vaccinations: Vaccines are available for certain STIs, such as human papillomavirus (HPV) and hepatitis B. Speak to your healthcare provider about vaccination options.

c. Open Communication: Communicate openly and honestly with your sexual partners about your sexual health and STI testing history.

d. Use Condoms: Consistent and correct condom use can significantly reduce the risk of contracting many STIs.

e. Limit Sexual Partners: Reducing the number of sexual partners can lower your risk of exposure to STIs.

4.3 Enhancing Sexual Pleasure and Communication

Prioritizing sexual pleasure while ensuring yoni health is essential for a satisfying intimate experience. Here are some tips for enhancing sexual pleasure and maintaining yoni well-being:

a. Lubrication: Use water-based or silicone-based lubricants during sexual activities to reduce friction and enhance comfort.

b. Communication: Open and honest communication with your partner about desires, boundaries, and any discomfort is crucial for a pleasurable and respectful sexual experience.

c. Post-Sex Hygiene: After sexual activities, urinating and cleansing the genital area with warm water can help prevent urinary tract infections (UTIs) and maintain yoni hygiene.

d. Regular Check-ups: Schedule regular gynecological check-ups to monitor your sexual health and discuss any concerns with your healthcare provider.

Prioritizing sexual health and safety not only enhances your intimate life but also contributes to overall physical and emotional well-being. In the following chapter, we will explore the impact of diet and lifestyle factors on yoni health and ways to manage stress for improved sexual health.

Chapter 5

Dietary and Lifestyle Factors

Diet and lifestyle choices have a significant impact on yoni health and overall well-being. By making informed decisions regarding nutrition, hydration, and stress management, women can promote a healthy and balanced yoni environment. In this chapter, we will explore the influence of diet on yoni health, the importance of staying hydrated, and effective stress management strategies.

5.1 The Impact of Diet on Yoni Health

A well-balanced diet plays a crucial role in maintaining optimal yoni health. Certain foods can contribute to a healthy yoni environment, while others may disrupt the yoni microbiome and increase the risk of infections. Here are some dietary factors to consider:

a. Probiotics: Consuming foods rich in probiotics, such as yogurt, kefir, sauerkraut, and kimchi, can help support the growth of beneficial bacteria in the yoni microbiome.

b. Prebiotics: Foods high in prebiotic fibers, such as garlic, onions, and bananas, can nourish the beneficial bacteria in the gut, which may indirectly impact yoni health.

c. Hydration: Drinking an adequate amount of water daily helps maintain overall body hydration, including the yoni tissues.

d. Sugar and Refined Carbohydrates: Diets high in sugar and refined carbohydrates can lead to imbalances in the yoni microbiome, potentially increasing the risk of yeast infections.

e. Antioxidant-Rich Foods: Foods rich in antioxidants, such as berries, leafy greens, and nuts, support overall immune health, which is essential for preventing and fighting infections.

5.2 Staying Hydrated and Its Effect on Yoni Moisture

Proper hydration is essential for maintaining healthy yoni tissues and promoting yoni moisture. When the body is adequately hydrated, the yoni tissues remain supple and well-lubricated, reducing the risk of discomfort and irritation. Aim to drink plenty of water throughout the day to stay hydrated.

5.3 Managing Stress and Its Impact on Yoni Health

Chronic stress can negatively impact yoni health, as well as overall physical and emotional well-being. High-stress levels may lead to hormonal imbalances, reduced immune function, and an increased risk of yoni issues. Here are some stress management strategies:

a. Exercise: Engage in regular physical activity to release endorphins and reduce stress.

b. Meditation and Mindfulness: Practice meditation, deep breathing exercises, or mindfulness techniques to promote relaxation and reduce stress levels.

c. Time Management: Organize your schedule and set realistic priorities to reduce feelings of overwhelm.

d. Support System: Reach out to friends, family, or professional support when dealing with stressors.

e. Hobbies and Leisure: Engage in hobbies and activities that bring you joy and relaxation.

By adopting a healthy diet, staying hydrated, and managing stress effectively, women can create a positive impact on their yoni health and overall quality of life. In the following chapter, we will discuss personal care products and their effects on yoni health, including the importance of choosing safe and suitable products for intimate care.

Chapter 6

Yoni Steaming: The Ancient Practice and Its Benefits

Yoni steaming, also known as yoni steaming or yoni detox, is an ancient practice that has been used by various cultures for centuries. It involves sitting over a bowl of steaming water infused with herbs, allowing the steam to rise and make contact with the yoni and surrounding areas. This traditional practice has recently gained popularity as a holistic approach to yoni health and self-care. In this chapter, we will explore the historical background of yoni steaming, its benefits, and important safety considerations.

6.1 Understanding Yoni Steaming

The practice of yoni steaming has roots in different cultures, including traditional Chinese medicine, Mayan healing traditions, and African herbal remedies. Historically, it was often used to address various gynecological concerns, such as menstrual discomfort, postpartum healing, and support for reproductive health.

During a yoni steaming session, a woman sits over a container of hot water infused with a blend of dried herbs, such as chamomile, rosemary, mugwort, calendula, or lavender. The steam rises and comes into contact with the yoni and vulvar tissues. The heat and herbal properties are believed to promote circulation, relax muscles, and potentially have a cleansing effect.

6.2 Historical Background of Yoni Steaming

Yoni steaming has been a part of traditional healing practices for centuries. Different cultures have utilized various combinations of herbs and techniques, often passed down through generations. While the scientific evidence supporting yoni steaming's specific benefits is limited, many women have reported positive experiences with the practice.

6.3 The Benefits and Risks of Yoni Steaming

Advocates of yoni steaming claim several potential benefits, although more research is needed to validate these claims. Some of the perceived benefits include:

a. Improved Circulation: The heat from the steam is believed to increase blood flow to the yoni and pelvic area, potentially aiding in tissue healing and revitalization.

b. Menstrual Support: Some women report reduced menstrual cramps and improved menstrual regularity after regular yoni steaming.

c. Postpartum Healing: Yoni steaming is believed to support postpartum healing and help tone the pelvic floor muscles.

d. Emotional Well-being: Many women find yoni steaming to be a relaxing and empowering self-care ritual that enhances emotional well-being.

However, it's crucial to consider potential risks and safety considerations:

a. Burns or Discomfort: Extreme heat or improper positioning over the steam can cause burns or discomfort. Caution should be exercised when practicing yoni steaming.

b. Disruption of Yoni Microbiome: Yoni steaming may disrupt the delicate balance of the yoni microbiome, potentially leading to infections or imbalances.

c. Unsuitable Herbs: The use of certain herbs may not be appropriate for every individual and could cause adverse reactions or allergic responses.

6.4 Precautions and Safety Guidelines for Yoni Steaming

If considering yoni steaming, it is essential to take the following precautions:

a. Consult with a Healthcare Professional: Before trying yoni steaming, consult with a qualified healthcare professional to discuss potential benefits and risks based on your individual health needs.

b. Use Safe and Suitable Herbs: Ensure that the herbs used for yoni steaming are safe and suitable for your specific health condition.

c. Avoid Extreme Heat: Be cautious not to expose yourself to extreme heat during the steaming process to prevent burns or discomfort.

d. Respect Individual Boundaries: Yoni steaming may not be suitable for everyone, and individuals should feel empowered to decide what practices align with their comfort and preferences.

In conclusion, yoni steaming is an ancient practice that has gained renewed interest in recent times. While it is essential to approach this practice with caution and respect for individual needs and safety, some women may find it to be a positive and beneficial addition to their self-care routine. As with any holistic approach, discussing yoni steaming with a healthcare professional is crucial to ensure it aligns with your specific health goals and concerns.

Some of the reasons women ought to steam.

a. Menstrual Support: Yoni steaming is believed to promote a healthy menstrual cycle by improving blood circulation to the pelvic area. Some women report reduced menstrual cramps and more regular periods after incorporating yoni steaming into their routine.

b. Vaginal Hygiene: Proponents claim that the steam can help cleanse the vagina and vulva, removing old residue and dead skin cells. This is believed to support vaginal hygiene and reduce the risk of infections.

c. Emotional Well-being: Yoni steaming is often considered a relaxing and meditative practice. The act of self-care and connecting with one's body can have positive effects on emotional well-being and stress reduction.

d. Postpartum Healing: Yoni steaming is sometimes used in postpartum care to support healing and toning of the pelvic floor muscles after childbirth. It is thought to aid in reducing inflammation and promoting overall recovery.

e. Uterine Health: Some proponents claim that yoni steaming can improve uterine health by stimulating blood flow to the area. This is believed to help with cleansing and toning the uterus.

f. Fertility Support: Yoni steaming is sometimes associated with fertility rituals and is believed to support reproductive health and fertility by promoting a healthy vaginal environment.

g. Connection with Femininity: The practice of yoni steaming is seen by many as a way to reconnect with their femininity and embrace their bodies' natural cycles and processes.

h. It's important to approach yoni steaming with caution and be aware of potential risks and limitations:

i. Safety Concerns: Yoni steaming involves exposure to steam and heat, which can cause burns or discomfort if not done carefully. Pregnant women, individuals with certain medical conditions, or those with sensitive skin should avoid or consult a healthcare provider before trying yoni steaming.

j. Vaginal Microbiome: There is concern that yoni steaming may disrupt the natural balance of the vaginal microbiome, potentially leading to infections or imbalances.

k. Limited Scientific Evidence: While many women report positive experiences with yoni steaming, there is a lack of rigorous scientific studies to support the claimed benefits.

In conclusion, yoni steaming is an ancient practice that has gained popularity in recent times. While some women find it to be a positive and beneficial addition to their self-care routine, it's essential to approach it with caution and respect individual boundaries. Consulting with a healthcare provider before trying yoni steaming is advisable, especially for those with specific health concerns.

Chapter 7

Personal Care Products and Their Effects

Personal care products play a significant role in maintaining yoni health and overall well-being. However, it is essential to be mindful of the products we use in the intimate area, as some ingredients may have adverse effects on yoni health. In this chapter, we will explore the importance of choosing safe and suitable products for intimate care, potential harmful ingredients to avoid, and natural alternatives that promote yoni health.

7.1 Evaluating Yoni Care Products in the Market

The market is flooded with a wide range of yoni care products, including soaps, washes, wipes, deodorants, and douches. While some of these products claim to promote freshness and cleanliness, they may contain harsh chemicals that can disrupt the natural pH balance and the yoni microbiome. When evaluating yoni care products, consider the following:

a. pH-Balanced Products: Choose products specifically formulated to match the natural pH of the yoni (around 3.5 to 4.5) to maintain a healthy acidic environment.

b. Fragrance-Free: Avoid products with added fragrances, as they can cause irritation and disrupt the natural scent of the yoni, which is essential for detecting any unusual odors that may indicate an issue.

c. Gentle Formulas: Look for products with gentle, non-irritating ingredients that are suitable for sensitive skin.

d. Hypoallergenic: If you have a history of skin allergies or sensitivities, consider hypoallergenic products that are less likely to cause adverse reactions.

e. Avoid Harsh Chemicals: Steer clear of products containing parabens, sulfates, phthalates, and other potentially harmful chemicals.

7.2 Potential Harmful Ingredients to Avoid

Certain ingredients commonly found in personal care products may be harmful to yoni health. Some harmful ingredients to avoid in intimate care products include:

a. Parabens: Used as preservatives, parabens have been linked to hormonal disruption and may interfere with reproductive health.

b. Sodium Lauryl Sulfate (SLS) and Sodium Laureth Sulfate (SLES): These foaming agents can strip the skin of its natural oils and disrupt the yoni microbiome.

c. Synthetic Fragrances: Artificial fragrances can cause irritation and allergic reactions, leading to discomfort.

d. Propylene Glycol: This chemical can cause skin irritation and may negatively affect the yoni pH balance.

7.3 Natural Alternatives for Yoni Care

Choosing natural alternatives for yoni care can be a safer and more beneficial option. Consider the following natural remedies and practices:

a. Warm Water: For daily cleansing, using warm water alone is often sufficient to maintain yoni hygiene.

b. Probiotic Foods: Incorporate probiotic-rich foods like yogurt and fermented vegetables into your diet to support a healthy yoni microbiome.

c. Coconut Oil: Organic, unrefined coconut oil can be used as a natural moisturizer for the vulvar area, promoting comfort and reducing dryness.

d. Herbal Rinses: Herbal rinses made from chamomile, calendula, or lavender can provide gentle cleansing and soothing effects.

e. Menstrual Cups or Cloth Pads: Consider using reusable menstrual cups or cloth pads to minimize exposure to potentially harmful chemicals found in disposable products.

By being conscious of the ingredients in personal care products and opting for natural alternatives, women can support their yoni health while reducing the risk of irritation or imbalances. In the next chapter, we will explore the importance of regular gynecological check-ups and self-examinations for early detection and prevention of potential issues.

Chapter 8

Gynecological Check-ups and Self-Examinations

Regular gynecological check-ups and self-examinations are essential for maintaining optimal yoni and reproductive health. These practices allow early detection of potential issues, prompt treatment of any abnormalities, and proactive management of overall well-being. In this chapter, we will explore the importance of regular gynecological check-ups, the benefits of self-examinations, and when to seek medical attention.

8.1 The Importance of Regular Gynecological Check-ups

Regular gynecological check-ups, also known as well-woman exams, are vital for women of all ages, regardless of whether they are experiencing any specific symptoms. During these visits, a healthcare provider specializing in women's health will conduct a comprehensive examination that may include:

a. Pelvic Examination: A physical examination of the external and internal reproductive organs, including the yoni, cervix, uterus, and ovaries.

b. Pap Smear: A test to screen for cervical cancer or detect any abnormal cervical cells.

c. Breast Examination: A check for any lumps, changes, or abnormalities in the breast tissue.

d. General Health Assessment: A review of overall health, medical history, and lifestyle factors that may affect reproductive health.

Regular gynecological check-ups allow healthcare providers to monitor any changes in yoni health, detect potential issues early, and provide appropriate guidance and treatment.

8.2 Conducting Self-Examinations at Home

In addition to regular gynecological check-ups, self-examinations can be empowering for women to monitor their own yoni health between visits. Here are some self-examinations women can perform at home:

a. Breast Self-Examination: Conduct monthly breast self-examinations to check for any lumps, changes, or abnormalities in the breast tissue. If any concerns are detected, consult a healthcare professional promptly.

b. Yoni Self-Examination: Familiarize yourself with the normal appearance and feel of your vulva and yoni. If you notice any new or unusual growths, changes in color or texture, or experience persistent itching, irritation, or discomfort, seek medical advice.

c. Menstrual Cycle Tracking: Keep track of your menstrual cycle to monitor regularity, flow, and any changes that may indicate underlying health issues.

8.3 When to Seek Medical Attention

It is crucial to seek medical attention promptly if you experience any of the following:

a. Unusual Yoni Symptoms: Persistent itching, burning, unusual discharge, or foul odor could be signs of infection or other issues.

b. Changes in Menstrual Pattern: Sudden changes in menstrual flow, irregular cycles, or heavy bleeding warrant medical evaluation.

c. Breast Abnormalities: If you notice any lumps, changes in breast size, or nipple discharge, consult a healthcare provider.

d. Pain or Discomfort: Any persistent pelvic pain or discomfort should be evaluated by a healthcare professional.

e. Abnormal Pap Smear Results: If you receive abnormal Pap smear results, follow up with your healthcare provider for further testing and guidance.

Remember that early detection and timely medical intervention can significantly improve outcomes for various gynecological conditions.

By prioritizing regular gynecological check-ups and performing self-examinations, women can take an active role in their reproductive health, ensuring early detection and prevention of potential issues. In the next chapter, we will address common yoni issues and practical tips to address them effectively.

Chapter 9

Common Yoni Issues and How to Address Them

While maintaining good yoni hygiene and overall health is essential, women may still encounter various yoni issues from time to time. Understanding these common concerns and knowing how to address them effectively can help promote yoni comfort and well-being. In this chapter, we will explore three common yoni issues - yoni itching and irritation, yoni discharge, and yoni odor - and provide practical tips on how to address them.

9.1 Yoni Itching and Irritation

Yoni itching and irritation can be uncomfortable and disruptive to daily life. Several factors can contribute to this issue, such as infections, allergies, or skin conditions. Here's how to address yoni itching and irritation:

a. Avoid Irritants: Avoid using products that may irritate the yoni area, such as scented soaps, detergents, and douches.

b. Wear Breathable Underwear: Choose cotton or other breathable fabric underwear to promote air circulation and reduce moisture retention.

c. Practice Good Hygiene: Maintain proper daily cleansing with gentle, pH-balanced cleansers, and avoid excessive scrubbing.

d. Consider OTC Creams: Over-the-counter antifungal or hydrocortisone creams may provide relief for mild irritation caused by yeast infections or skin irritations. Consult a healthcare provider before using any medication.

e. See a Healthcare Provider: If the itching and irritation persist or worsen, consult a healthcare provider to rule out any underlying infections or conditions that may require specific treatment.

9.2 Yoni Discharge: What's Normal and What's Not

Yoni discharge is a normal and healthy occurrence that helps to cleanse and protect the yoni area. However, changes in the color, consistency, or odor of yoni discharge may indicate an issue. Here's how to address yoni discharge:

a. Monitor Changes: Pay attention to any sudden changes in the color, texture, or smell of your yoni discharge.

b. Normal Discharge: Normal yoni discharge is usually clear or white, with a slight odor that is not unpleasant.

c. Abnormal Discharge: If you notice discharge that is yellow, green, gray, or has a strong, foul odor, it may indicate an infection, such as bacterial vaginosis or a sexually transmitted infection (STI).

d. Seek Medical Evaluation: If you experience abnormal discharge or any associated symptoms like itching or pain, consult a healthcare provider for proper diagnosis and treatment.

9.3 Dealing with Yoni Odor

Yoni odor is normal to some extent and can vary based on hormonal changes, menstrual cycles, or sexual activity. However, persistent or strong odors may be a sign of an underlying issue. Here's how to address yoni odor:

a. Maintain Good Hygiene: Regularly cleanse the external genitalia with water and a mild, pH-balanced cleanser. Avoid harsh soaps or douches.

b. Breathable Fabrics: Wear breathable, cotton underwear to promote air circulation and reduce odor caused by trapped moisture.

c. Avoid Tight Clothing: Tight clothing can trap moisture and increase the risk of odor. Opt for loose-fitting clothing when possible.

d. See a Healthcare Provider: If you experience persistent, strong, or unusual yoni odor, seek medical evaluation to rule out any infections or medical conditions that may require treatment.

It's essential to listen to your body and be proactive in addressing any yoni issues that arise. While some minor concerns may resolve with home care, persistent or severe symptoms should prompt a visit to a healthcare provider for proper evaluation and treatment.

In the next chapter, we will discuss the importance of nurturing yoni health during pregnancy and postpartum, including helpful tips for self-care during these transformative phases of a woman's life.

Chapter 10

Pregnancy and Postpartum Yoni Care

Pregnancy and postpartum are transformative phases in a woman's life that require special attention to yoni health and well-being. During pregnancy, hormonal changes and increased blood flow to the pelvic area can affect yoni health. After childbirth, the body undergoes significant changes, and proper care is essential for healing and recovery. In this chapter, we will explore the importance of nurturing yoni health during pregnancy and postpartum, along with helpful tips for self-care during these stages.

10.1 Pregnancy and Yoni Health

During pregnancy, the body goes through various changes that can impact yoni health. Some common concerns during pregnancy include:

a. Increased Discharge: It is normal to experience increased yoni discharge during pregnancy, which helps protect the yoni and cervix from infections.

b. Yoni Dryness: Some women may experience yoni dryness due to hormonal fluctuations during pregnancy. Using a water-based lubricant can provide relief during sexual activity.

c. Yeast Infections: Pregnant women may be more suscep-
tible to yeast infections due to hormonal changes and
increased glucose levels in yoni secretions.

d. Pelvic Floor Health: Practicing Kegel exercises can help
strengthen the pelvic floor muscles, which can be beneficial during pregnancy and prepare for childbirth.

e. Avoiding Irritants: During pregnancy, it's essential to
avoid using harsh soaps, douches, or scented products
that can disrupt the delicate balance of the yoni microbiome.

10.2 Postpartum Yoni Care

After childbirth, the body needs time to heal and recover.
Proper postpartum yoni care can aid in the healing process
and promote comfort. Consider the following postpartum
care tips:

a. Rest and Recovery: Allow your body ample time to rest
and heal after childbirth. Avoid strenuous activities and
lifting heavy objects during the initial weeks.

b. Perineal Care: Gently clean the perineal area with warm
water after using the toilet. Consider using a peri-bottle
to rinse the area and pat it dry with a clean towel.

c. Soothing Measures: Warm sitz baths can provide soothing relief for any discomfort in the perineal area. Adding
Epsom salts or herbal infusions can enhance the healing
benefits.

d. Supportive Underwear: Choose comfortable, breathable
underwear that offers support and allows air circulation.

e. Pelvic Floor Exercises: Gradually resume pelvic floor exercises (Kegels) to strengthen the muscles and promote
bladder control.

f. Intimacy: If you have any concerns about resuming sexual activity after childbirth, consult with your healthcare provider. Using water-based lubricants can be helpful if experiencing yoni dryness.

10.3 Seeking Professional Support

Throughout pregnancy and postpartum, it's essential to maintain open communication with your healthcare provider. Regular prenatal check-ups during pregnancy allow for monitoring of yoni health and addressing any concerns. After childbirth, postpartum check-ups can help ensure proper healing and address any issues related to yoni health.

Remember, every woman's pregnancy and postpartum experience is unique. It's essential to listen to your body, seek support when needed, and prioritize self-care during these transformative stages of motherhood.

In the concluding chapter, we will summarize the key points discussed throughout the book and emphasize the importance of adopting a holistic approach to yoni health for overall well-being.

Chapter 11

Aging and Menopause

As women age, the body undergoes natural changes, including those related to the reproductive system. Menopause, the cessation of menstrual periods, marks a significant milestone in a woman's life. Understanding the effects of aging and menopause on yoni health is essential for maintaining comfort and well-being during this transition. In this chapter, we will explore the impact of aging and menopause on yoni health, common concerns, and practical tips for self-care.

11.1 The Impact of Aging on Yoni Health

As women age, the yoni tissues undergo changes due to hormonal fluctuations and reduced estrogen levels. Some effects of aging on yoni health include:

a. Yoni Dryness: Lower estrogen levels can lead to yoni dryness, which may result in discomfort during sexual activity.

b. Thinning of Yoni Tissues: Reduced estrogen can cause the yoni walls to become thinner and more fragile, making them prone to irritation and inflammation.

c. Weakening of Pelvic Floor Muscles: Aging can lead to weakened pelvic floor muscles, contributing to issues such as urinary incontinence and pelvic organ prolapse.

d. Decreased Lubrication: Aging can affect the body's natural lubrication, leading to discomfort during sexual activity.

11.2 Menopause and Yoni Health

Menopause, which typically occurs between the ages of 45 and 55, marks the end of the reproductive years. During menopause, estrogen levels decline significantly, leading to various changes in the body, including:

a. Yoni Atrophy: Reduced estrogen can cause the yoni tissues to become thinner, drier, and less elastic, a condition known as yoni atrophy.

b. Hot Flashes: Menopause is often associated with hot flashes, which can lead to increased body temperature and sweating.

c. Mood Changes: Hormonal fluctuations during menopause may contribute to mood swings, anxiety, or irritability.

d. Sleep Disturbances: Some women experience sleep disturbances, such as difficulty falling asleep or staying asleep, during menopause.

11.3 Practical Tips for Self-Care during Aging and Menopause

Self-care is essential for promoting yoni health and overall well-being during aging and menopause. Consider the following tips:

a. Use Water-Based Lubricants: During sexual activity, use water-based lubricants to alleviate yoni dryness and enhance comfort.

b. Pelvic Floor Exercises: Continue practicing pelvic floor exercises to maintain muscle strength and support bladder control.

c. Seek Medical Advice: If experiencing yoni dryness, discomfort, or other concerns, consult with a healthcare provider for appropriate treatment options.

d. Stay Active: Engage in regular physical activity to promote overall health and well-being.

e. Healthy Diet: Adopt a balanced diet rich in nutrients to support general health and hormonal balance.

f. Manage Stress: Implement stress management techniques such as meditation, deep breathing, or yoga to cope with menopausal symptoms.

g. Regular Check-ups: Continue regular gynecological check-ups and follow-up visits to monitor yoni health and address any concerns.

11.4 Embracing the Aging Process

Embracing the aging process and menopause as natural phases of life is essential for women's emotional well-being. It is an opportunity to focus on self-care, prioritize health, and celebrate the wisdom gained through life experiences.

By nurturing yoni health and adopting a holistic approach to self-care during aging and menopause, women can embrace this new phase of life with confidence and grace.

In the concluding chapter, we will summarize the key points discussed throughout the book and emphasize the importance of embracing and prioritizing yoni health as an essential aspect of overall well-being at every stage of life.

Chapter 12

Empowering Your Yoni Health Journey

Throughout this book, we have explored various aspects of yoni health and the importance of prioritizing self-care at every stage of a woman's life. Empowering your yoni health journey involves understanding your body, being proactive in seeking care, and embracing a holistic approach to well-being. In this final chapter, we will summarize the key takeaways and provide empowering steps to support your yoni health journey.

12.1 Key Takeaways

Let's recap the key points discussed in this book:

a. Yoni Health is Essential: Prioritize your yoni health as a crucial aspect of overall well-being. Practicing good hygiene, choosing suitable products, and regular check-ups contribute to a healthy yoni environment.

b. Menstrual Care: Select appropriate menstrual products, practice good hygiene, and be attentive to your menstrual cycle. Address menstrual discomfort proactively and manage your period with care.

c. Safe Sex Practices: Emphasize safe sex practices, use contraception effectively, and prioritize regular STI testing to maintain sexual health and safety.

d. Diet and Lifestyle: Adopt a balanced diet, stay hydrated, and manage stress to promote optimal yoni health and overall wellness.

e. Yoni Steaming: Understand the ancient practice of yoni steaming, its benefits, and potential risks. Always exercise caution and seek professional advice if considering this practice.

f. Gynecological Check-ups: Attend regular gynecological check-ups, perform self-examinations, and seek medical attention promptly if you notice any concerning changes or symptoms.

g. Pregnancy and Postpartum Care: Nurture your yoni health during pregnancy and postpartum, allowing proper healing and recovery after childbirth.

h. Aging and Menopause: Embrace the natural changes that occur with aging and menopause, prioritize self-care, and seek medical guidance for any menopausal symptoms or concerns.

12.2 Empowering Steps for Your Yoni Health Journey

To empower your yoni health journey, consider the following steps:

a. Knowledge is Power: Educate yourself about your body and yoni health. Stay informed about common issues and best practices for self-care.

b. Listen to Your Body: Pay attention to any changes or discomfort in your yoni health. Trust your instincts and seek medical advice when needed.

c. Advocate for Yourself: Be an active participant in your healthcare. Ask questions, seek second opinions, and ensure your concerns are heard and addressed.

d. Prioritize Self-Care: Make time for self-care activities that promote yoni and overall health, such as regular exercise, stress management, and relaxation techniques.

e. Build a Support Network: Surround yourself with a supportive network of friends, family, and healthcare professionals who can provide guidance and encouragement on your journey.

f. Embrace Changes: Embrace the changes that come with different life stages. Empower yourself with knowledge and support to navigate these transitions with confidence.

g. Celebrate Your Body: Appreciate your body and all that it does for you. Celebrate your femininity and the uniqueness of your journey.

Remember that every woman's yoni health journey is unique. Your journey may include ups and downs, but by empowering yourself with knowledge, self-care, and proactive healthcare, you can confidently navigate the path towards optimal yoni health and overall well-being.

As you continue on your yoni health journey, always remember that you have the power to prioritize your health, seek support when needed, and embrace the wisdom that comes with caring for yourself holistically.

BONUS

THESE ARE SOME REASONS WOMEN SHOIULD STEAM THEIR YONIS.

Check our store out today for your YONI Needs.

Cleansing

The uterus is a self-cleaning organ. Every month it grows a brand new uterine lining and every month it sheds that lining unless you become pregnant. Cleansing herbs support the body's natural ability to release the old lining so that something new can be build up in it's place.

Hydrating

Water is the often forgotten essential nutrient of life. We take for granted how much water our body really needs in order to function. Certain herbs are known as kidney tonics.

Disinfecting

The genitals have their very own microbiome, colonies of friendly bacteria that live symbiotically with us. If these bacteria become unbalanced (likely stemming from an imbalance in your gut) certain herbs have properties that help balance the microbiome.

Blood building

After each period your body needs to replenish the blood that was lost. Blood is rich in nutrients and blood building herbs support the body's ability to create new blood cells.

Digestion Support

It may seem weird to include digestive support in a Yoni Steam herb recipe, but all health issues start in the gut! In Traditional Chinese Medicine these herbs are known to promote chi circulation. Chi is your life force, your energy. Adding chi and digestion supporting herbs brings vigor and vitality to the body.

Decrease Bleeding

These herbs are known as anti-hemorrhagic. Uterine fatigue is not a medical condition, rather a collection of signs that the uterus lacks strength to complete a full, normal cycle. Short cycles, where your period comes too early, frequent spotting and spontaneous bleeding, are all signs of uterine fatigue and can be supported by steaming with anti-hemorragic herbs.

Women in this state are generally very sensitive to stimulation by herbs. If you experience any of the signs of uterine fatigue, I strongly recommend purchasing a pre-formulated herbal blend or working with an herbalist rather than creating your own yoni steam recipe, unless you are an experienced herbalist yourself.

Uterus Strengthening

Women prone to signs of uterine fatigue also benefit from herbs that strengthen the utuers. In Traditional Chinese Medicine these are known as chi tonors. They help to tone and strengthen the chi, or life force of the body.

Follow us on IG at : havenhisher

About the author

Dr. Ava Eagle Brown is a remarkable individual, serving as the CEO and founder of TheMangoGirlPublishing -(Bookz-biz). She is a multi-award-winning International Speaker, Author, and Transformation Mindset Business Coach. With a global reach, Dr. Ava coaches, trains, and delivers inspiring speeches to empower others in shifting their mindsets, leading to transformative changes in their lives and businesses, ultimately impacting their bottom-line positively.

Residing in the UK for over twenty years, she now divides her time between London and Jamaica, where she envisions making her permanent home. Dr. Ava is the talented author of several books, including "The Mango Girl Publishing," captivating readers with her compelling stories and insights. Beyond being an accomplished author, she is an independent book publisher, dedicated to bringing diverse voices and perspectives to the literary world.

Through her impactful work and inspiring journey, Dr. Ava Eagle Brown continues to leave a lasting legacy, motivating countless individuals worldwide to embrace change, growth, and empowerment. Her passion for uplifting others is evident in the transformation she facilitates through her coaching, speaking engagements, and publishing endeavors.

To contact her email: business@avaeaglebrown.com

Instagram at : havenhishers

"Empowering women through top-tier intimate care products and services, and elevating men's performance. Join us for confidence and wellness.